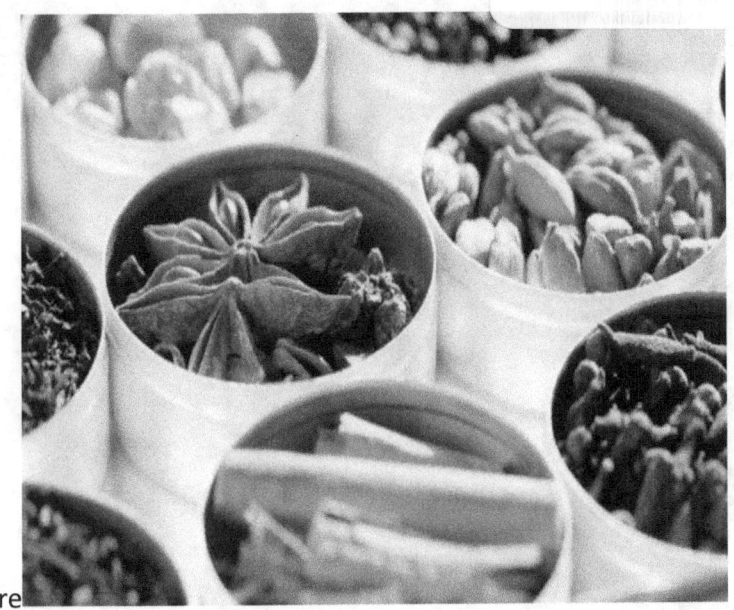

re

HERBAL REMEDIES FOR STRESS

Herbal and Aromatherapy Recipes You Can Make

Demetria Clark

Herbal Remedies for Stress

Herbal and Aromatherapy Recipes You Can Make

Demetria Clark

Note to the Reader: This is an informational guide, a recipe book. It is not meant to prescribe, diagnose or replace medical care and treatment. This book is not intended as medical advice, and should not be viewed as such. There are potential risks associated with herbs and essential oils. Because of this, the author, writer, publisher and/or distributors of these book are not responsible for any adverse reactions or effects associated with any information and recipes in this book. If you have a medical condition or want to use herbal remedies speak to your care provider first. Review all information, research each herb and essential oil before use and do not use something that you feel is not safe or in the proper application.

First Printing: 2014
©Demetria Clark
ISBN-13: 978-1500457822
ISBN-10: 1500457825
www.heartofherbs.com

All images contained are used with a licensing agreement with Shutterstock. Other images are the property of Demetria Clark and Andrew Clark.

DEDICATION

To anyone and everyone who has ever suffered the effects of stress in their daily lives. Hopefully we can offer you some herbal tips to assist you.

CONTENTS

ACKNOWLEDGMENTS

I want to thank all of our students and supporters who through the years
have really become part of our family.

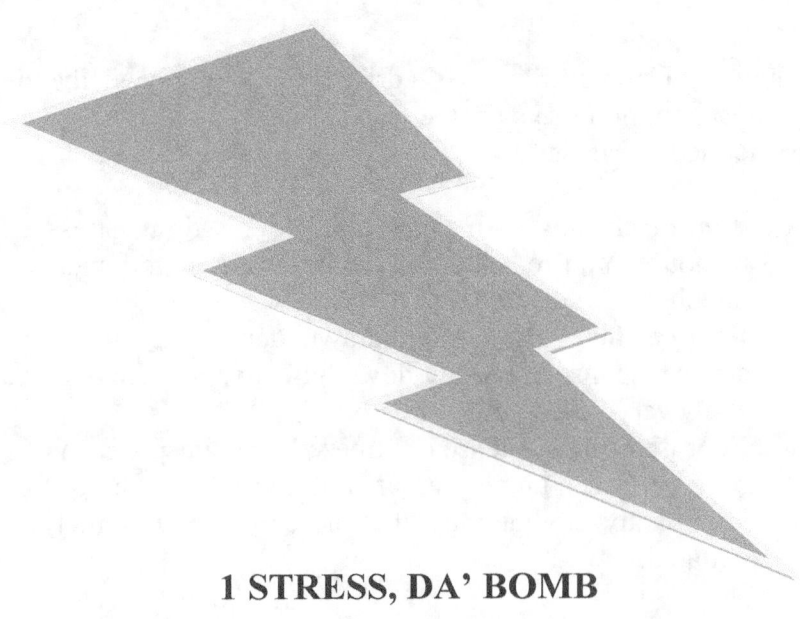

1 STRESS, DA' BOMB

Our stress levels can affect every aspect of our lives. The body reacts and changes to stimulus, and these are in physical, mental and emotional responses. A normal part of life is stress.

When events happen around you, your stress levels are the reaction to these events. Some events cause acute stress and others cause chronic stress. Our reactions to these events affect us every day, in our everyday reactions.

Stress is Da' Bomb on our lives. Stress makes us irritable, angry, tired, grumpy, and anxious emotionally. Physically it can cause aches and pains, diarrhea or constipation, nausea, dizziness, chest pain, rapid heartbeat, loss of sex drive and frequent colds. Getting a handle on stress levels can really make a difference in your everyday life.

Psychologist Connie Lillas uses a driving analogy to describe the three most common ways people respond when they're overwhelmed by stress:

- **Foot on the gas** – An angry, agitated, or "fight" stress response. You're heated, keyed up, overly emotional, and unable to sit still.
- **Foot on the brake** – A withdrawn, depressed, or "flight" stress response. You shut down, pull away, space out, and show very little energy or emotion.
- **Foot on both** – A tense or "freeze" stress response. You become frozen under pressure and can't do anything. You look paralyzed, but under the surface you're extremely agitated.[1]

Some tips for relieving stress are:

Sunbathe: Regular time outside in the sun. Take a few minutes a day to sunbathe. 15-20 minutes 2 times a day will make a huge difference. Your vitamin D levels will increase and your overall outlook should also improve.

Take Time: Take time to read, meditate, and find time to relax for 20 minutes a day. If you have a tight work schedule then do the sun and relaxation at the same time. Take the time to take a relaxing bath.

Eat a Healthy Diet: Worry less about being "fat" and more about being healthy. Eat foods a close to nature as you can. Choose options that have the least amount of processing. If you eat meat, dairy or eggs, choose higher quality options. I know these things can cost more, but hitting the farmer's market, local farm shops or growing your own can assist with some of the costs. Opting to eat in 2 times a month or changing your coffee shop routine can often

[1] Smith, M. Segal, R. & Segal, J. (n.d.). Stress Symptoms, Signs, & Causes. *Stress Symptoms, Signs & Causes: Effects of Stress Overload.* Retrieved July 8, 2014, from http://www.helpguide.org/mental/stress_signs.htm

assist saving up a good chunk of cash. Visiting Asian markets are a great way to get healthy options on the cheap also.

Sleep: Get enough sleep. Make sure you get solid and restful sleep. Turn off the television, radio and put your chat notification and cell phones to sleep. You do not need to be online all night. I know this sounds obvious to some, but even my most astute and aware clients have a hard time insuring they get enough sleep and down time. Down time or sleeping the appropriate amount, and needing it, is not a sign of weakness.

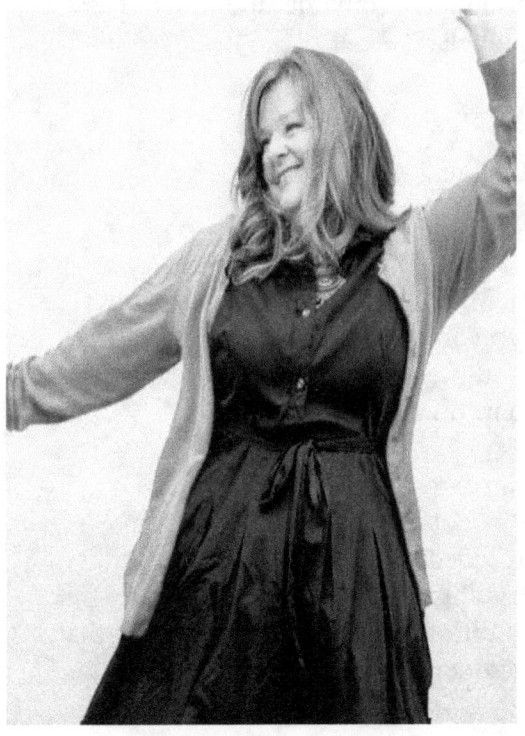

Take a nap if you need too. Give yourself permission to take care of yourself. You deserve it. If you have small children at home then try to rest when they do. Find and use more efficient strategies to get housework and obligations taken care of.

If you fall asleep whenever you watch a movie or read a book it may mean you need more down time.

Move! Shake it! Move your tushie: Make sure your take the time to move ever hour. Squats over the toilet, twists, dancing, touch your toes, go up and down on your tippy toes. Make some unexpected movements to get the blood flowing and reinvigorate yourself.

Get yourself hooked into a regular activity. Take up golf, swimming, yoga, kickboxing, disco roller skating and anything else you have always wanted to do. Give yourself this gift. Many resources are available. Learn about your local parks, botanical gardens, playgrounds, etc... And visit them more.

I love singing and dancing. When I am the most stressed out you will find me singing at the top of my lungs every time I get into the car.

Think about what makes your life less stressful. Is it a song? A scent? A cup of tea?

Hopefully I can share some herbal and aromatherapy tools to assist you with lessening your stress levels.

Disclaimer

All of herbs, essential oils and recipes are just that recipes. It is up to you the reader to research them to make sure you will not have a reaction. Some are not safe if you are pregnant or nursing, others may cause issues with high blood pressure, or other issues. Do your due diligence and be a smart user and consumer.

The information presented in this book is provided for informational purposes only, it is not meant to substitute for medical advice or diagnosis provided by your physician or other medical professional. Do not use this information to diagnose, treat or cure any illness or health condition. If you have, or suspect that you have a medical problem, contact your physician or health care provider for advice and counsel.

2 SAFETY IS THE NAME OF THE GAME

HOW TO USE THIS BOOK
Listen to Yourself
Believe and reconnect with your instincts. You know when something is not working for you, listen to your inner voice. If you do not like how something feels, do not use it.

Patch testing skin
A patch test can be done by dabbing, with a cotton swab, a little on a small area on your skin, inner arm, or the back of your knee, and if a reaction occurs then it could be an indication for not using the blend.

Patch Testing the Environment
Before you use something to clean fabric, carpet, tile, porcelain, fiberglass, linoleum, etc... Please test the cleaning formula on a small area. Sometimes discoloration can occur, even though they are generally safe. It is important you test your environment before using. Just because something works for me, or someone else, does not mean it will work for you, or your surfaces. Someone else may have a cotton rug, and yours is wool, many variables exists, so please be aware of this.

Know What is Inside
Know what you are using. Check Latin names, also called Botanical or Scientific names, and look up the herb or essential oil before you use anything. Don't just assume that something will work for you, just because it is listed in a book. Like anything else, remedies, solutions, etc... Are all individual. You are in charge of your own body, so if any of these recommendations cause an interaction or reaction stop using it.

Safety Tips for Essential Oils

1.   Make sure what you are buying is an actual essential oil. Read the label. The ingredients should say for example- Sweet Orange (Citrus sinensis) Essential Oil- Nothing more. Sometimes an essential oil in a store may contain a carrier oil that should also be clearly marked with the oils name. If you are buying a pure essential oil then that is all the product should contain.

2.   Make sure you as the user properly use essential oils. Do not ingest, or apply neat if you want to use safely during pregnancy. This overall is a great rule to follow. I have been using essential oils for over 25 years and I never apply essential oils neat, even "safe ones". This is because I am never sure how an oil will act or react on any person at any time or even myself at any given time. Being careful doesn't mean I don't have faith in the healing attributes, but it means I am aware of the overall power of the plants.

3.   Some oils over time can cause sensitization or allergic reactions. So making sure you never use undiluted oil and alternating the oils you use can assist in preventing that. If an allergic reaction occurs remove the oil the best you can, milk or cooking oil can assist with that. The essential oil bonds to the fat in the milk or oil and then you can shower to assist in further removal. Soaking a washcloth or paper towel in oil or milk and applying to the affected area followed by a bath or shower can assist with removing the oil. I always suggest clients' patch test before using any oil.

 • *Simple patch test instructions, again, said another way, it is that important.*- Apply 1-2 drops of the diluted essential oil to the crease of your elbow, then cover the area or keep it dry for 24 hours. If a reaction occurs then this oil may not be the one for you. Remember that even if an oil does not cause a reaction for you it may for someone else.
 Less is more- In our current world we think more is better, but in reality often that is not the case and it is not the case when

working with essential oils. One thing you can always do is use less. If a dosage is 5 drops, see if you get the same results with 2. You do not need to use or make a formula any stronger than you need. Some people get the same results from 1 drop as another does with 5.

Do your homework

Before you buy, and before you use, read about the oil, or make sure it is the one you want. Research the oil, smell it from a few sources, and find the oil you want. Many health food stores, herb shops and essential oil suppliers often have display oils you can smell. Take advantage of these displays and learn about the different scents of these oils. Do not ask a company for free samples. For some reason in the alternative health field we seem to think it is okay to ask for free samples, consultations, lessons, etc.. This is not a healthy path to continue on. Most people will not ask a plumber, mechanic, doctor, bookstore, health food store, etc.. for free product and services, so please be respectful of the businesses you are working with, just the same way.

Smell the oils

If purchasing oil at a physical location smell the oil samples and make sure you like it. If the oil's scent really turns you off, then find an alternative, listen to yourself. You can always revisit that oil, you did not like at a later date and see if you have the same experience. Often I have at times smelled an oil and thought, "Augh.. gross" and re-smelled a few months later and loved it, or at least felt differently about the oil. I believe these reactions really have something to do with where we are at a given moment, and listening to what our bodies need. Luckily in almost all cases you can find an alternative oil to support your needs.

Remember that essential oils are flammable. Use caution and care when using them near an open flame, such as a candle diffuser. Read all instructions well on diffusers, vaporizers, candle dispersers, and other types tools for essential oil dispersal.

Take care to avoid getting essential oils in or on mucus membranes, eyes and genitals. If you get essential oils in your eyes flush them with milk or oil and seek appropriate medical care and advisement. If you get essential oils on your genital areas rinse with oil or milk. You can make a milk sitz bath for vaginal exposure.

STOP

If irritation occurs   using the essential oil blend.

Use appropriate caution when using essential oils with infants, children, pregnancy and elder care.

Never use essential oils internally. Some resources may offer instructions on how to do so, but unless under appropriate care, but since this is a self-care book we are advising no internal use.

Some of these recipes may seem familiar. Some have been included in previous teachings, course materials, lectures and articles online and in my classes. Some of them are from as far back as 1990, some have even been rewritten and placed online. That can occur with recipes, especially with the internet, I have found whole pages of my recipes online word for word, some dating back to original printings in 1998.

Enjoy yourself

Allow yourself to mess up, try again. Herbalism and Aromatherapy are not exact sciences, like all health care options, each person reacts differently and responds differently.

You Are in Charge

As an adult, you are in charge and responsible for your own health. I use herbs exclusively in the treatment of my children, my husband and myself, through illnesses, pregnancy and breastfeeding. I have never been faced with a situation in which herbs have not worked for us, even in acute situations that have required hospital assistance, herbals have assisted greatly in after care and pain management. As an adult your health care choices are up to you, in most situations you can make informed decisions. There can be times when you sense something might not be working effectively for you, or when you feel uneasy about, for example one more round of antibiotics. It is these times more often than not that clients come to me with questions and a desire to try what they consider a more natural and gentler form of treatment. I advise them to be sure to consult their physicians or health care practitioners before changing treatment, and to educate themselves, via books, courses or consulting an herbalist, before they begin to prescribe remedies to themselves or stop medications or plans their doctors have them on. Most care providers what to do what is best for the patient and they will work with you. Unfortunately in our current medical climate it may not feel that way, but that we have to remember is not the care provider per se but the system they work in, a system we all have to work in to make better.

Essential Oil, Extraction, Storage and Safety

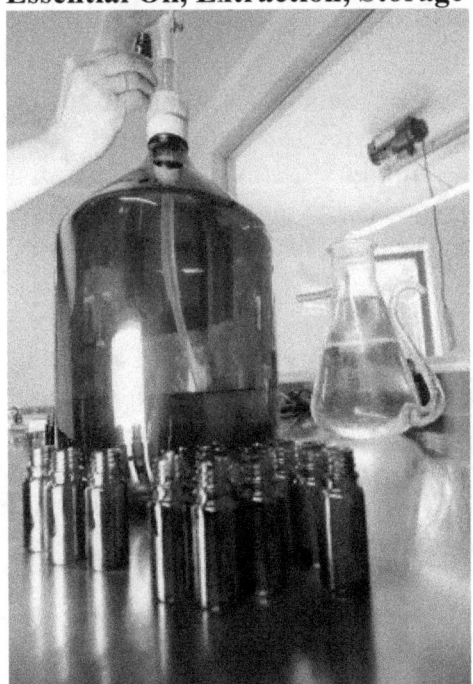

The following is information about essential oils to include hazardous essential oil list. These are particularly dangerous and not appropriate for use, especially by women who are pregnant, nursing or postpartum. These are all the essential oils and not the herbs themselves. A lot of essential oils are not safe for pregnancy are not on this list, this is a list of oils that in general are not safe for use. When an oil is considered not safe for pregnancy, it usually has to do with having an "Emmenagogue" effect, meaning they stimulate menstrual flow, contraction stimulation, they have abortifacient properties (can cause a miscarriage) or can cause harm to the mother or fetus.

Some essential oils have "reputations" for causing one health side effect or another. Many can't be proven with scientific studies or research, but until we have another batch of information we will have to go on the research and information of the day.

Extraction Methods of Essential Oils

These are many different ways to make an extract and essential oil from a plant.

Absolute

An absolute, is not considered a true essential oil, but a classification of its own, but you will often see absolutes being sold side-by-side with essential oils. An absolute is obtained through chemical solvent extraction, and not a true essential oil. Generally the solvent used is alcohol and the alcohol is removed with vacuum extraction. The most common absolutes are Jasmine (Jasminum grandiflorum), Rose and at times Sandalwood (Santalum album).

Enfleurage

This is an ancient manner of extracting essential oils using odorless fats and oils to absorb the critical scent qualities from plants. This method is not as commonly used in modern essential oils. It was most commonly used with plants like Jasmine (Jasminum grandiflorum), Honeysuckle, and other highly scented fatty flowers.

Expression

This method of extracting essential oils from plant material, physically expresses the complete oil from the plant. An example of this is citrus peel when you peel an Orange (Citrus sinensis) you bend the rind, expressing the essential oil from the peel, the liquid the squeezes out is essential oil. This method is also known as cold pressing oils, or cold pressed extractions.

Hydrosol

A hydrosol is the name for the water left after a steam or water distillation of an essential oil. It is mainly water with only a very small amount of water soluble plant constituents. Generally because a hydrosol is mainly water you can use them directly on the skin. Research each one though before using.

Distillation

The most common method of obtaining essential oils is through steam distillation. Remember moonshine stills? This offers a similar idea on how the process occurs. The water is heated to boiling point, and then the steam passes through fresh plant material that has been placed on a rack above the boiling water. The steam and the pressure of the steam is carefully controlled. When the steam passes through the plant material it causes the cell walls of the plants to swell and break down this allows the release of the essential oil. Then the essential oil vapor and water pass through a condenser that cools the steam and the oil into a liquid. The liquid is collected and separation occurs. Most essential oils are lighter than water and collect, or float to the top of the water and they are then siphoned off. Oils that weigh more than water sink to the bottom of the collector and they are then separated.

If you are interested in purchasing your own essential oil distiller you can buy them online, prices vary from about $300.00 to $5000.00 dollars. You can even find instructions online for stills you can make on your own.

Essential Oil Quality
Choosing an essential oil or an essential oil company to purchase from can be daunting. Some basic tips are as follows:

Follow your nose, it may take some time and experience but smelling essential oils is one of the first tips I give for choosing an essential oil. Does the oil smell like the plant part it is distilled from? Can you smell a chemically smell? Can you smell "fillers"? If you can smell chemicals or fillers you may want to pass those oils over.

Read the labels, the ingredients should just be essential oil, unless you are purchasing a blend or diluted blend. We wary of labels that have the words "nature identical oil," "fragrance oil," or "perfume oil." These words may be a sign of that what you see is not a pure, single essential oil. On the label you should be able to see the common name and the Latin plant name, make sure the Latin plant name is the essential oil you desire. Some plants have different varieties as essential oils. For example Orange (Citrus sinensis) oil could be Sweet Orange (Citrus sinensis) (Citrus sinensis) or Bitter Orange (Citrus aurantium). Although that example wouldn't be common it is an example.

Most reputable essential oil companies will offer labeling with more information, instead of less. They want you to know

you are purchasing a quality product.

Be leery of terms like "therapeutic grade", "medical grade" or "aromatherapy grade" essential oils. We have no formal standards for these terms and they are being used: Until a standardized description and official grades are made that are universally respected I will tend to not use them to access an oils quality.

Many great brands may have these descriptions or sales and marketing slogans, but overall they are just that descriptions.

As a selling tactic. As a basis for sale, individuals will usually spend more for terms like these whether the quality warrants it or not.

Or as a way to distinguish a product. Although this is not necessarily wrong, as the consumer you need to know that this is not a formal recognition gained to assure quality or purity of the oil. Many in the industry are trying to get rid of these terms because they are confusing to consumers, and some feel misleading.

Fortunately we have no shortage of quality essential oil suppliers and most will answer your questions and welcome feedback from customers. Here are some shopping tips to assist you with your essential oil purchasing.

> *Most essential oils have a year plus shelf life, so that investment is good for at least a year.*

When buying oils make sure it is in a dark bottle, amber is the darkest and I feel really the best, but you can find violet, cobalt and green. They need to have an orifice reducer, not a dropper. Droppers erode from the essential oil and allow air to enter. You need to in addition avoid oils in plastic or clear bottles. Most reputable essential oil companies sell in 4oz. bottles and smaller. Generally a 1 oz. bottle will last you quite a while.

Essential oils are not cheap. Look around online and in stores to see what a baseline price is and if the price is too good to be true, then it probably is. In a brief search I found that most organic Peppermint essential oils for an ounce varied from $11-25.00. If you are planning on buying a few oils you can start with smaller sizes and later you can purchase the larger sizes of the oils that you use on a regular basis. So for $100-150.00 you can get a decent assortment of essential oils. I know that this may seem like a lot of money, but to put it in perspective it is not going out to dinner 1-2 times at a nice restaurant in a year or giving up a few activities over the course of a year. You can also buy the oils as needed spreading out the investment. At the end of the book you will find a resource section for essential oils companies that do mail order.

When purchasing online make sure the oils are not all the same price. When you purchase essential oil in bulk to rebottle, they are not all the same price, so selling them for the same price is a little suspect, at least in my opinion. Not all cars can be priced the same, eggs have different prices in the market, and so basic business practices makes this practice of pricing unsustainable.

When at a store looking at a sample, if you put a drop on your finger it should feel clean and not to oily. Essential oils are not true oils like a fruit seed or vegetable oil, so they should not feel greasy. Some of the thickest, darker oils like Vetiver (Vetiveria zizanoides) or Patchouli (Pogostemon cablin) can have a thicker oil feeling than something like Lavender (Lavendula officinalis) or Sweet Orange (Citrus sinensis).

Essential Oil Storage

Essential oils can last from 1 year to many years. Some factors to consider are the type of oil and how they are stored. Here are some simple storage guidelines.

Store all essential oils in a cool dark place. Direct sunlight or light at all will rapidly speed up oxidization and promote breakdown within the oil. I found at an antique store a small

Often darker colored essential oils have a longer shelf life than lighter colored oils. Lighter colored oils often evaporate faster in air than darker.

cabinet from an apothecary shop that works well.

Make sure all oils are in dark bottles with a tightly closing cap. Droppers are not acceptable for storage. The bubble rubber will disintegrate in the vapors of the essential oils. If you use a dropper with the oil, you can purchase them separately and wash them between use or purchase extras and have one for each oil. Most oils come with orifice reducers which are small inserts that allow only one drop to leave the bottle at a time.

Shelf life- Most essential oils have a shelf life of two years. Patchouli (Pogostemon cablin) and Sandalwood (Santalum album) can last a few years longer and Tea Tree (Melaleuca alternifolia), fir and Pine (Pinus sylvestris)last about 18 months and citrus oils usually 1 year, longer if they were distilled closer to the time of purchase.

HERBS

BUYING HERBS- Always buy organically grown herbs. Try to buy local herbs whenever possible. Herb growers are everywhere, you just have to look around.

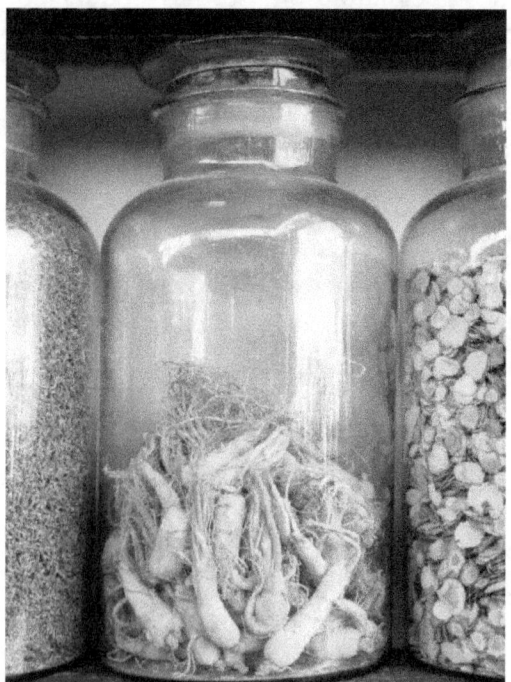

Most large herb companies fumigate their plants because pests could wipe out their entire stock. Many companies also have begun to irradiate their herbs to kill pests, especially if they are coming from overseas. Herbs face importation issues just like produce does. Buying herbs from a distributor who uses overseas suppliers increases your chances of getting irradiated and fumigated products. While I understand the need to protect stock and follow laws governing import, I do because of these regulations purchase herbs as locally as possible. Many companies are trying to implore safer and more natural means of stock protection.

Using chemically free herbs is as important as eating chemically free foods, but not just for our personal health. When we choose organics, we promote sustainable farming and biodiversity, help reduce pollution, protect the soil and water, and make work safer for farmers and farm workers. Think how much better you will feel, not just physically but emotionally, when you nourish your body and your family with clean, honorably produced food. When we make choices that protect our environment, we are also making choices that protect our bodies.

Buying locally supports your neighbors and smaller farms. Shop for organic herbs at your farmer's market, this is also a great place to get starter plants for your garden, vegetables, fruits and herbs. Get to know the people who grow them. When I buy garlic or Echinacea plants from the farmer down the road, I know I'm getting fresh and potent garlic, and strong local Echinacea, and that will do its job in my remedies.

Buying locally fosters community, directly makes a difference in your local economy and lessens your carbon footprint.

If you can't buy locally, seek out organic herbs and herbal products at natural-food stores—usually in the bulk section—or from specialty retailers. Research your sources.

GROWING YOUR OWN HERBS

Gardening books may feature elaborate herbal knot gardens that look complicated and intimidating, but the fact is, herbs are easy to grow. And they can be grown just about anywhere there is good soil, sunshine, and water (and maybe a little compost once in a while). You can grow herbs in a small plot in the yard; in a corner of your garden; or in pots on your porch, patio, or kitchen window sill.

Basic information about growing herbs can be found in almost any gardening book. You can also ask local gardeners, and herb vendors at the farmers' market. These resources can really help you in learning what grows well in your area. Many will have excellent tips that work in your area, how to work your soil and what varieties do really well in your area. When we moved to NC it was the first time I had a garden with lots of clay, having neighbors who gardened and a good relationship with the farmers at the market really was helpful in getting tips for my region. I had gardens in Vermont, New York and Switzerland, but all climates and soils are different, so having insider information is so beneficial.

When planting your herb garden, try to plant from seeds as much as possible. This saves money, of course, and it also teaches you about gardening and what grows well in your area. Don't be concerned with straight-as-an-arrow row planting or pulling every last weed. Gardening is supposed to be a fun stress reliever. Just trust in the process and allow yourself to observe the journey from seed to harvest.

Wildcrafting simply means gathering plants from the wild—from fields, meadows, mountainsides, natural areas, pastures, or anywhere you can legally pick herbs. If you are not on public lands, request permission from the property owner. This a good way to give herbalist a bad name in a community. Many people skip this step, and don't ask, that is a great way to get someone mad at you. Most people in my experience are tickled to let you pick wild plants from their pastures, fields and woods, as long as you are polite, respectful to them and the land. You never know you may also make a new friend.

Never harvest more than you can use, and never deplete a local plant stand. I often tell my students not to pick more than 10 percent of an existing herbal stand or patch. (However, that percentage can vary depending on the size of the patch.) Other people in the community may also want to harvest the plants. Also consider that animals and insects rely on plants for food, pollination, and other necessities.

Do not pick protected plants. Find out which plants are protected in your area and use a good field guide to identify them.

Just because a plant appears to be plentiful does not automatically mean you can pick it. And a plant that is not protected in one area may be protected in another, so find out which plants are protected wherever you wildcraft. If in doubt, don't harvest the plant. Information about protected plants can be found on state wildlife websites (most will have a link to this information) and the USDA website at http://plants.usda.gov/threat.html.

Ways to Use Herbs
Tea

Tea is the use of water and herbs to make an extraction. Water in the case of tea is the solvent. Teas are used for refreshment and as beverages. You can also make a medicinal tea. Medicinal teas are made the same way as infusions and decoctions.

Infusion

Infusions use the more fragile parts of plants, like leaves and flowers. There are few exceptions to this and Valerian (Valeriana officinalis) is one root prepared as an infusion because of its high volatile oil content, in a blend it can still be part of a decoction though, if other roots are in the blend. This involves pouring boiling water over the plant matter and allowing the matter to infuse. A medicinal infusion steeps for 20 minutes - overnight.

I really like to let my infusions steep for a generous amount of time. I like to allow steeping to occur for about an hour, others only steep for 20 minutes, and it is a personal choice. If it is an herbal tea I really want to enjoy hot I add it to a thermos, or insulated cup to keep it warm.

It is really important to me that they are medicinally potent because I suggest teas for so many tonic and medicinal uses.

Brewing Guide

Type of Tea	Temperature	Steeping Time
Black Tea	212 F or Boiling	3-5 Minutes Steeping Time
Green or White Tea	170-185 F	3-5 Minutes Steeping Time

Oolong	185-210 F	4-7 Minutes Steeping Time
Herbal Teas	212 F or Boiling	5-10 Minutes
Herbal Infusions		At least 20 minutes. Preferably at least an hour.

These are just guidelines, but it is important to be patient and allow tea to properly steep. If it becomes cool and you want it warm, just rewarm before drinking.

Decoctions

This is the method used to get the plant healing constituents from more tenacious plant material such as bark, root or nuts. This is simmered gently with the herb in the water for 20 minutes.

For pre-blended roots and leaves the decoction is the preferred method of preparation. The same goes for a decoction: I really like to let my infusions steep for a generous amount of time.

It is really important to me that they are medicinally potent because I suggest teas for so many tonic and medicinal uses.

Amounts of herb used for decoction or infusion: 1 tablespoon dried herb per cup of water, or two tablespoons fresh herb per cup of water. Teas can be made by the quart and refrigerated for daily consumption.

I often make large jars of tea to have around all day to drink from or to pour from. Infusions and decoctions when made in bulk need to be stored in the refrigerator, and then only for 48 hours at the most.

Nervous System Tea-simple tea recipe
1 part Valerian (Valeriana officinalis) root
1 part Skullcap (Scutellaria lateriflora) herb
1 part Hops (Humulus lupulus) flower
1 part Spearmint (Mentha spicata) leaf
Honey to taste
Prepare as an infusion
You can drink 3-6 cups a day.

Liniments

A liniment is an herbal extraction that is rubbed into the skin. Liniments are used for sore muscles, strains, arthritis, and inflammations or the muscles, ligaments and tendons. A liniment is usually herb and a solvent such as alcohol, vinegar or oil.

To make a liniment for sore muscles for example one would place 4 oz. Of Peppermint in a jar that is 16 oz. Also add 4 oz. Of Eucalyptus. Add a pint of alcohol, or vinegar. Do not use rubbing alcohol, use Vodka. Place in a nice dry place for 14 days and shake twice a day. Then use on the affected areas. You can also add a few drops of essential oil like Rosemary, Peppermint or Eucalyptus.

For an instant liniment for muscle pain is this

½ cup alcohol, vodka will work.
1-teaspoon Peppermint (Mentha piperita) essential oil, eucalyptus or Rosemary (Rosmarinus officinalis) oil. You should first try using less essential oil at first and find the amount that works for you.

Extracts

Extracts can be very easy to make, and a very convenient way to take herbs. First off place as much herb as you want into a glass jar. Then add your alcohol. I usually add three fingers higher than the herb (dried herb) and two fingers higher than fresh herb. Close the jar and allow it to sit in the sunlight for a few days to soak in the solar healing power of the sun and then put it away until done. If it is macerating during a full moon put it outside to gather the moon's energy also. I also allow my extracts to sit for over four months. Many people only allow them to sit for a few weeks to a month. This is not something I advise. I believe an extract should be made to offer the most healing benefits.

Some herbs as we will learn are best made into teas rather than extracts. An easy formula to follow for making herbal medicine is the simplers' method, this method is based on ratios, and the measurements are referred to as "parts". For example 3 parts Alfalfa (Medicago sativa), 1 part nettle, 2 parts raspberry, is a very common 3:1:2 synergy. This simple way of measurement lets you make your formulation in any volume you wish, whether ounces, tablespoons, cups, liters, or grams for example. This is a traditional way to formulate with herbs.

Always store your extracts in glass, in a dry, dark spot.

Example- 40% alcohol is 80 proof. All of the alcohol percentages are just baselines, you may find some things work better for you in different ways, please find the way that works best for you.

Then the liquid is poured through a cloth, such as layers of cheesecloth, a kitchen towel with a loose weave or very fine sieve or colander. The herbs that remain are squeezed thoroughly to remove as much of the fluid from them as possible. Extracts can be made of single herbs, or herbal blends, depending upon your needs. Some herbalist run the extracted herbs through a juicer and strain to achieve the best extract they can, or press the extract to get all they can from it. These are all fine ways of doing it, it really is a matter of preference.

It is time-honored traditional magic to begin your extracts on the eve of the new moon, and strain on the full moon, so that the waxing powers of the moon extract the greatest amount of therapeutic agents from the herbs.

Extract Alcohol Percentages

A good way to decide how much alcohol to use is this

35-40% for leaves and flowers

40-60% for barks, roots and seeds

90% for Kava Root, Kava is best fat extracted.

Tinctures

A tincture is a diluted extract, traditionally. The tincture is diluted 5x, from the original extract. Unfortunately the term tincture is often misused to describe and extract, so your product would then be weaker. In many cases individuals selling extracts call them tinctures because this is the common name for the process.

In other instances you want a lower percentage solution and a tincture may be exactly what you need.

Poultice

A poultice is similar to a compress except that plant parts are used rather than liquid extraction. Mash or crush fresh plant parts. Heat them in a pot over boiling water or mix them with a diminutive amount of boiling water. Apply the pulp directly to the skin, as hot as can be tolerated, holding it in place with a gauze bandage. When using dried herb, first powder it and make a paste with 1 tablespoon of powdered herb and a little boiling water or hot cider vinegar, organic. If the paste is likely to irritate the skin, apply it between two layers of cloth. I suggest wool. I secondly suggest fresh wool that has been gently cleaned and is still full of Lanolin. I have a few bags around at all times so I can use the wool I want. Some is barely washed and other pieces are really clean, it depends on what I am, treating with a poultice. Poultices are generally more active than compresses. They are used to arouse circulation, appease aches and pains or draw impurities out through the skin, depending on the herb chosen.

A hot water bottle held against the poultice may keep the heat in for as long as needed. Once it cools, it should be changed and another, as hot as tolerable, applied in its place. Please make sure you don't burn anyone or yourself. Also remember to change the poultice whenever it cools.

Plaster

Prepare the herb parts as for either a steamed or pulped poultice, but place the warm mass of pulverized herbs between two layers of cloth before applying to the desired area. Depending on the herbs used, plasters can be left in place for an extended period of time, even overnight.

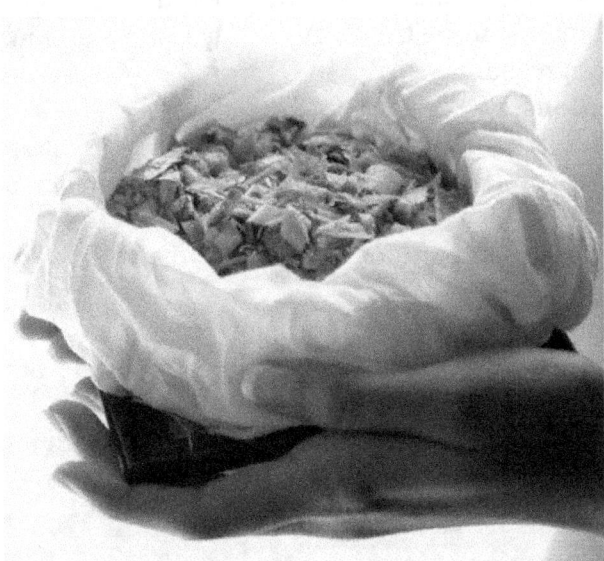

Compress

A compress is made by soaking a piece of clean cloth (such as linen, cotton, or gauze) in a decoction or infusion and applying it as hot as can be tolerated to the affected area. When the compress has cooled, it can be soaked again in the reheated liquid and reapplied until the condition has been relieved. Compresses can also be applied cold. I make cold ones for my son's boo-boos. One of my favorite compresses is one that contains Arnica (Arnica montana) and Plantain (Plantago major) for bruising. My sweet sons are extremely rambunctious and I find this one is used an awful lot. I have also made compresses from extracts in water. I find that these not only work extremely well but they are easy to use on the go.

Alternate instructions

Wash your hands thoroughly and soak a soft cloth or clean flannel in the liquid mixture, which consists of 2 cups (500 ml) infusion or decoction, or 1 ½ Tablespoon (25 ml) tincture in 2 cups (500 ml) water. Wring out the excess liquid. Before applying, rub a little oil on the affected area to prevent sticking. Place the compress against the affected area. For pain and swellings, secure the compress with plastic film and safety pins and leave for up to 1 to 2 hours. Re-apply as required. You can also layer wool in the plastic to keep the compress warm.

You can also make a compress from essential oil, water and a cloth. Soak a cloth in a bowl of water with a few drops of essential oil, such as Tea Tree (Melaleuca alternifolia) or Lavender (Lavandula angustifolia).

Salve

A salve is a firm beeswax and oil combination that is for external application. Salves can be applied by smoothing on your skin, it will gently spread and melt into the surface of your skin. Salves can be for emotion and physical issues.

Simple Salve Instructions

You need an oil, olive oil or infused oil such as Plantain (Plantago major), Comfrey (Symphytum officinale) or Calendula (Calendula officinalis).

You can estimate the proportions based on the following equivalents.

One pint of oil will need about 1 1/2 ounces of beeswax, or one ounce of oil will need about 1/2 teaspoon of beeswax. There are about 5 teaspoons of beeswax in an ounce.

You then need to heat the oil with the beeswax and mix until all of the wax is melted. Then you add your herbs and essential oils and pour into containers. If the salve is too hard re-melt and add more oil, and if too soft re-melt and add more wax. Instead of wax you can use a vegetarian wax or coconut oil.

Inhalation

An inhalation is when one uses steam to administer herbs or essential oils. The person inhales the steam into their lungs and nose and mouth. This method is great for head colds and sinus ailments.

Inhalation (Portable method)

1 or 2 oz. Bottle or vial

Few grains of large rock salt.

Few drops essential oil.

For clearing nasal passage you could use Rosemary (Rosmarinus officinalis), Eucalyptus, or Peppermint.

For calming oneself you can use Lavender (Lavandula angustifolia), Clary Sage, for a mild uplifting stimulation is Sweet Orange (Citrus sinensis), Grapefruit (Citrus paradisi) or Mandarin Essential oil.

Over The Bowl Inhalation

Pour boiling water/ very hot water into a bowl. Add a drop or two of essential oil or a few tablespoons of herbs. Then place a towel over your head and bowl and inhale the steam. Please remember not to get your face too close to the hot steam and please be careful not to knock over your bowl.

In the Shower Inhalation

Plug up the tub and start your shower, when a small amount of water has collected add your essential oil and shower. The water will activate the essential oil and provide for inhalation.

Kerchief Inhalation

One can add a few drops to their Kerchief and smell the kerchief when one needs a pick me up.

You can also inhale herbs using a humidifier or vaporizer by adding a few drops to the water. Or you can place a pot of water on the stove add water and herb or essential oil and allow the water to simmer. This is great for children because it is portable and extremely simple to use.

Storing Herbs

Storage containers should be airtight, and dark.
Ideally herbs should be stored in sterilized, dark glass containers with airtight lids.

Label containers

Label all containers with the name of the herb and the date. Glass is the best containers to use. Many restaurants love to donate large glass jars. Many jars can be reused like large pickle, relish, maraschino cherry, etc... Labeling is extremely important, a lot of plants can look and smell alike dry and be complete opposites for healing.

Make sure you also label using the scientific name and the date the herb wash put into the container.

Temperature & Humidity

Store dry herbs at room temperature.
Store in a cool, dry place away from sunlight, moisture, and dust. This is really important.

Shelf life
Leaves, flowers, roots, and other herb parts

Keep for about a year after harvesting in cool place. Store in sterilized, dark glass containers with airtight lids. (May also store in new brown paper bags, which must be kept dry and away from light.) Paper bags inside of Tupperware like containers also work.
Frozen herbs

Herbs frozen in freezer bags keep up to 6 months. You can do this with a lot of your cooking herbs and take out pieces when you want and it tastes like you used fresh herb.
Infusions

Make fresh daily. Store in refrigerator or cool place. They will last a day or two. You can also make in Popsicles for easy child application.
Decoctions

Consume within 48 hours. Store in refrigerator or cool place. You can also make in Popsicles for easy child application.
Tinctures, syrups, and essential oils

Keep for several months or years. Store in dark glass bottles in a cool environment away from sunlight. Store syrup in the refrigerator for up to 1 month, unless a preservative is present such as glycerin or alcohol. Essential oils will evaporate; you must keep them tightly sealed.

Ointments, salves creams, and capsules

These can keep for several months. Store in dark glass jars. You can use hard plastic containers, but they can sometimes degrade, so please use high quality plastic. You can extend the life of creams or anything that combines oil and water by storing them in the refrigerator.

Capsules should be stored as soon as they are made, so they can enter storage in the freshest manner. Anytime left out in the open air will aid in them degrading.

Ointments should be stored in airtight jars and pots. Because they often have a large amount of essential oil, make sure the pots are airtight.

Remedies	Shelf Life
Dried herb material properly stored	1 year
Frozen herbal material	6 months
Infusions and Decoction- refrigerated	48 hours
Extracts/Tinctures properly stored	1-20 years
Essential Oils	1-10 years
Ointments, Salves, Balms	6 month- 2 years
Creams and Lotions, anything with a combination of fat and water.	3-6 months
Capsules	3-6 months

Guidelines for Using Herbs Safely

Here are some rules of thumb for how and when to safely take herbal medicines. Always check with a qualified health practitioner before taking an herbal supplement.

1. Buy organically grown herbs.

2. Discontinue taking any herb immediately if you feel it disagrees with you (you could be allergic to a medicinal herb just as you could a drug). Even if you know you don't like something but you can't find why you don't like it, discontinue use, your body is trying to tell you something. Listen to your body.

3. Be certain the herb has been properly identified as the herb you think it is. This is especially important for using bulk herbs. LABEL!

4. Pay close attention to recommended dosages for different herbs and properly adjust dosages for children, elders and those with weak constitutions.

5. Many herbal teas and herbs in food are safe for daily use over time, but stronger forms of herbs including extracts should not be used for more than brief periods without a naturopathic doctor or trained herbalist's supervision. Some herbs cannot be used under certain circumstances. Learn about your body and your health.

6. If you have a chronic medical condition, use herbs under medical supervision. Some herbs will interact with medication and they should not be used without the proper education and supervision.

3 STRESS BATH RECIPES

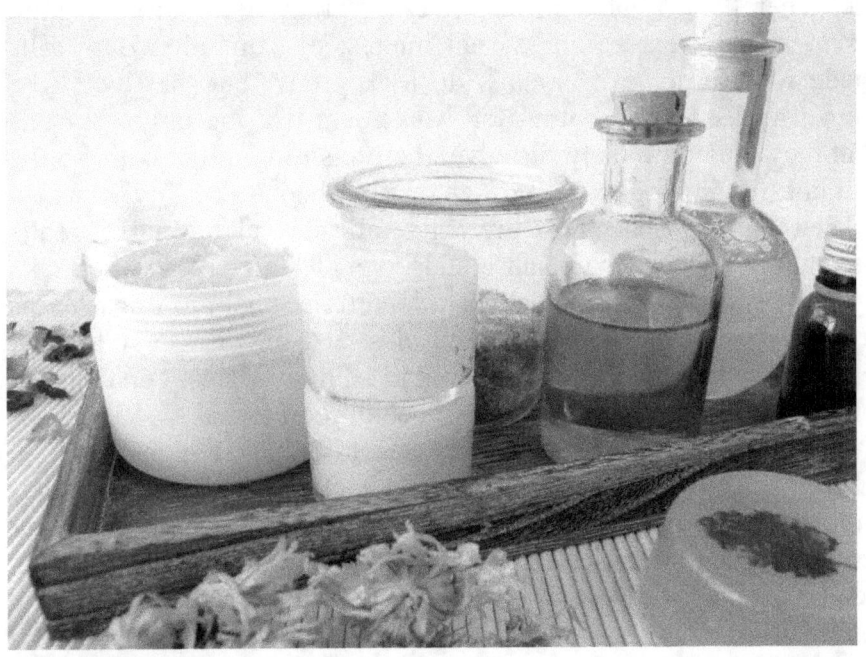

BATH SALTS

The use of salt in healing stretches back to the beginning of time. The healer Hippocrates encouraged his companion healers to offer as a cure for many issues immersion in sea water. The ancient Greeks continued this, and it is still considered healthy to sea bathe. Dr. Charles Russel published "The Uses of Sea Water" in 1753. Many healing modality texts have spoken of the benefits of sea bathing for hundreds of years. Taking the waters, hydrotherapy, are all common types of using baths to heal.

Essentially bath salts are salt, different types of salt and scent. If you want to add a little moisture to your bath you can add a teaspoon oil, like olive, sesame, coconut well mixed in. If you want them to have bubbles, you can add soap flakes, or liquid soap. You can add ground herbs that are powdered, oatmeal and herbal teas to make therapeutic baths.

Many of these sea salt recipes have been part of my recipe collection for years. I have been using and teaching these recipes since 1998.

The following is a list of commonly available salts that are often used when making bath salts. Sea salts and Dead Sea salts are generally available in a variety of grain sizes. Mixing grain sizes can add texture and visual interest to bath salts. Bath salts made with larger salt crystals do look pretty, but they will take longer to dissolve in bathwater. Make sure if using larger crystals that they are completely dissolved before sitting in the bath, so the salt doesn't feel jagged and rough on your bum.

Sea Salts: Sea salts are mineral-rich "all purpose" salts commonly added to bath salt blends. Next to Epsom salts, sea salts are the most inexpensive salts available. They help to draw toxins from the skin and soothe sore muscles. Sea salts are easy to find, most Asian markets sell them in 5 and 10 pound bags, you can also find sea salts in grocery stores and health food stores.

Dead Sea Salts: Dead Sea salts generally have a higher mineral concentration than conventional sea salts. Dead Sea salts can assist in relieving muscular aches and pains, reduce stiffness after exertion, relax muscles and relieve skin complications such as acne, eczema and psoriasis. Dead Sea salts are often coveted by sufferers of skin issues because they sooth these kinds of skin issues so well.

Epsom: Epsom salts are the most affordable and readily available salts, you can get them in most grocery or drug stores. They are often used to help ease muscle tension and joint discomfort. Epsom salts are a fine white crystal powder that can be purchased in any drugstore. They are hydrated magnesium sulfate. Soaking in these salts is soothing to sore muscles because the salts are mildly astringent. They are also used as a laxative (when taken internally) and as an anti-inflammatory soak. Epsom salts are often the go-to salts for athletes, the salts sooth and relax tired and worn out muscles.

Exotic Salts: Other more exotic salts such as Hawaiian Red Sea Salts (Alaea), Black Sea Pink Salts, and Icelandic Geo-Thermal Brine Salts are also available.

These salts generally are more expensive, but their coloration, texture and therapeutic properties are highly sought after. Having bathed in the Red Sea I can attest to the healing power of the salts, they made my skin feel so soft and rejuvenated.

I really feel that I understood the real healing power of sea salt bath after I had my first son. Relaxing and floating in the bath was heavenly. But I was wrong, I truly experienced the power of salt water when I was floating in the Red Sea, I was as peaceful as I had ever been in my life. I am no salt water novice, I have swam in the Pacific Ocean, Atlantic, Caribbean Sea, Red Sea, Mediterranean Sea, Labrador Sea, Gulf of Alaska and the Gulf of Mexico.

You can by looking online find stores that essentially just sell sea salts and types of sea salts. Some are soft, some are crystalline and others are almost a moist powder. You will eventually find the salt that will become your favorite.

In all of these recipes EO means essential oils. In some cases I write it out and in others I just use EO.
All bath salts should be stored in air tight containers and properly labeled. If a reaction occurs, sometimes it can happen, remove your body from the bath and rinse off immediately.

Bath Salts- Basic Base Recipe
2 parts Sea Salt any type, your choice.
2 Parts Borax, Mineral Salts
1 part Epsom Salts
1/4 part powdered herb matter like Lavender (Lavendula officinalis) or Rosemary (Rosmarinus officinalis) (optional)
A few drops essential oil, like Lavender (Lavendula officinalis), Rosemary (Rosmarinus officinalis) or other oils like Rose (Rosa damascene), Sandalwood (Santalum album), Palmarosa (Cymbopogon martini), Rosewood (Aniba rosaeodora) and other essential oils you like.
Essential oil guideline 15 drops per cup of bath salts. As you learn what you prefer you can modify the Essential oil amount.

Most baths require between a ½ cup to one cups of prepared salts.

Bath Salt Recipes
Soothing Bath Salts
2 pounds Epsom salts
1 pound sea salt
1/2 pound Dead Sea salts
1 1/2 cups vegetable glycerin
1/4 ounce Lavender (Lavendula officinalis) Essential Oil
1/16 ounce Helichrysum (Helichrysum angustifolia) essential oil
1/16 ounce Geranium (Pelargonium graveolens) essential oil
1/4 ounce baking soda
Mix all dry ingredients together. Place EOs in glycerin and let set for one hour. Add glycerin mixture in salts and knead well. Let set for 24 hours and knead again. Use 1/4 to 1/2 cup per bath.

DeStress It Away
2 cups Epsom salts
2 cups baking soda
10 drops Lavender essential Oil
10 drops Clary Sage essential oil
Mix well and add to your bath. Use 1 cup per bath.
This is good for de-stressing and mental relaxation.

Stress Buster
2 cups Dead Sea salt or other sea salt
8 drops of Geranium essential oils
8 drops Ylang-Ylang essential oil
8 drops of Lavender essential oil
This is good for deep relaxation.

Muscle Relaxing Bath
2 cups sea salt
1 cup mineral salts
7 drops Black Pepper (Piper nigrum) essential oil
7 drops Cypress (Cupressus sempervirens) essential oil
Combine in an airtight container and use as needed. ½ cup at a time. This recipe is good for stress manifesting in muscle tension. These recipes can easily be doubled or tripled as needed.

Mint Bath
1 cup fresh spearmint simmered
½ cup Oatmeal
5 drops Peppermint essential oil
Simmer the finely ground oatmeal and fresh spearmint for 15 minutes in 5 cups of water.
Strain, add the essential oil and pour into bath. Make sure the bath is finely dispersed.

Vanilla Relaxing Bath
Scrape a Vanilla Pod- scrape into the salt.
1 cup Sea Salt
1 cup Epsom Salt
5 drops Sweet Orange essential oil
5 drops Lavender essential oil
   Stir the vanilla into the salts and allow the mixture to sit for at least 24 hours.
Add the essential oils and mix well.

BATH TEAS
Bath teas are teas that are made in large pots allowed to cool and then added to the bath. Generally a bath tea is made in a stock pot. I like to add the whole pot of tea, strained to my baths. The amount of herb used is individual. Many people just use a tablespoon or two of each for ease. I generally like to use total one cup of herbs per gallon of water. Add the herbs to the water, bring to a boil and allow to cool and strain.
Generally for a bath I use between a ¼ -1/2 per herb.
2 cups of herb total per bath.

Calming Tea Bath
Equal parts of, for instance for enough for one bath use
Chamomile Flowers
Lavender Flowers
Rose Petals
Blend all together and make as a tea. 1 cup per two gallons of water. Strain and add to the bath. You can also add orange peel or Lemon Balm (Melissa officinalis) also.

Stress Relief Tea
Spearmint Leaf
Rosemary
Lavender Flower
Sage
Blend all together and make as a tea. 1 cup per two gallons of water. Strain and add to the bath.

Stress Relief Tea II
Lemon Verbena
Lavender Flowers
Calendula (Calendula officinalis) Petals
Lemon Balm
Blend all together and make as a tea. 1 cup per two gallons of water. Strain and add to the bath.

Head Space Centering Bath Tea
Equal parts of, for instance for enough for one bath use.
Chamomile
Lemon Balm
Linden Flower
Pinch of Rosemary.

Bath teas take a little prep, but you can premix the dried herbs for use later. You can also use fresh herbs.

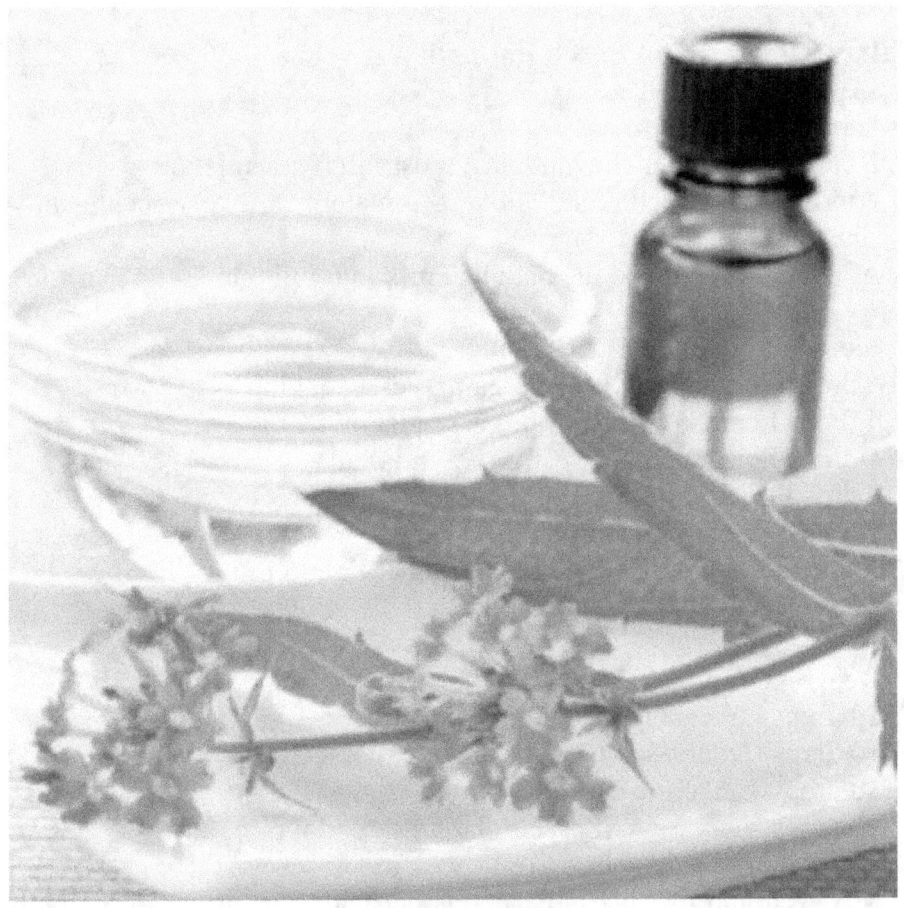

BATH OILS

Generally with bath oils all you need per bath is 1 teaspoon to 1 tablespoon of oil. A little oil goes a really long way. Make sure you mix the oil into the bath water, to disperse the oil and make sure you are careful when leaving the bath, the tub may be slippery.

Relaxing Oil
1/2 cup carrier oil
12 drops Sandalwood (Santalum album) essential oil
10 drops Orange essential oil
15 drops Clary Sage (Salvia sclarea) essential oil
Add a teaspoon or two to the bath.

Lavender Alcohol Based Bath Oil
1/2 cup Carrier Oil
1/8 cup vodka
20 drops Lavender (Lavandula angustifolia) essential oil
Pour in a glass bottle and allow it to mature for two weeks, gently shaking to mix every day.
Add 2 tablespoons to the bath and mix into full tub.

Sleepytime Bath Oil Blend
5 drops Bergamot (Citrus bergamia) essential oil
4 drops Lemon (Citrus limon) essential oil
4 drops Pine (Pinus sylvestris) essential oil
2 drop Cedarwood (Cedrus atlantica) essential oil
5 drop Mandarin essential oil
½ cup Grapeseed, Borage seed or other light oil.
Mix the essential oils into the

DeStress and Rest Bath Oil
20 drops Lavender (Lavandula angustifolia) essential oil
10 drops Cedarwood (Cedrus atlantica) essential oil
30 drops Tangerine essential oil
10 drops Clary Sage (Salvia sclarea) essential oil
1 cup of jojoba, hazelnut, sunflower, or Grapeseed oil
Mix well and use 1-2 tablespoons per bath. Or further dilute with at least another ½ cup of oil and use as a massage oil.

4 BODY SPRAYS

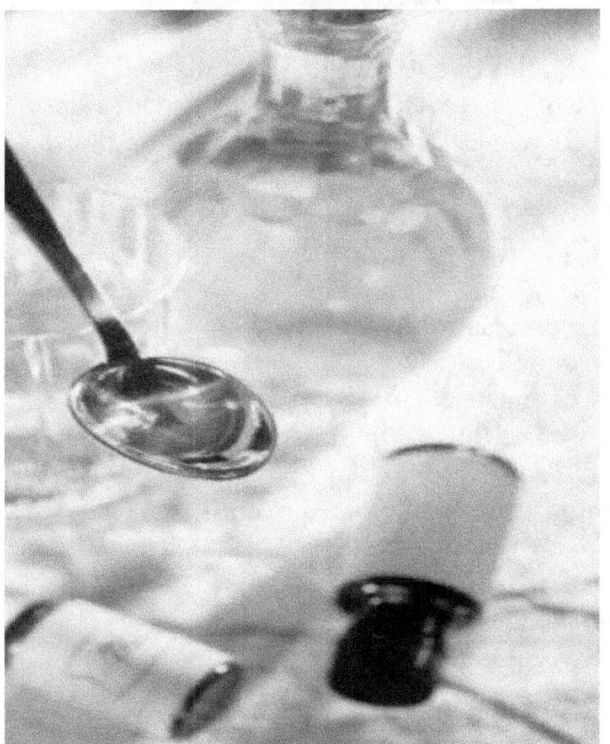

Body mists can be therapeutic, or used just as a fragrance for the body. Everyone has their own sense of smell and what they like in a fragrance. Feel free to alter and make the scent one you like.

All of the body mists listed here are all made to be dispersed in water. If you want you can add a teaspoon vodka for preservation. When using a body spray mist your skin, avoiding the face and genitals. If using as a room mist, you just gently spray a few mists into the air. If you are making a body oil you can add the essential oils to a carrier oil instead of water. Use the same amount of oil, as you would water. So if the recipe requires 2 oz. water, replace it with 2 oz. of carrier oil.
You can also use body sprays as room spray.

Relaxation and Rest Body Spray

15 drops Lavender (Lavendula officinalis) essential oil
10 drops Roman Chamomile (Matricaria chamomilla) essential oil
15 drops Clary Sage (Salvia sclarea) essential oil
Add to a 4 oz. mister.
Add the essential oils to the mister bottle and then add the water, cap and shake well. Mist your body, or the area around you. I like this blend for when I come home from a long birth and I need to relax.

Super Chill Body Spray

20 drops Clary Sage
15 drops Lemon Balm
5 drops Patchouli
Add to a 4 oz. mister.
Add the essential oils to the mister bottle and then add the water, cap and shake well. Mist your body, or the area around you. I like this blend for when I really need to chill out.

Lavender Citrus Spray

20 drops Lavender essential oil
20 drops Sweet Orange essential oil.
Add to a 4 oz. mister.
Add the essential oils to the mister bottle and then add the water, cap and shake well. Mist your body, or the area around you. I like this blend for clearing the air, refreshing and relaxing a room.

Princess Panic

10 drops Lavender essential oil
10 drops Mandarin orange essential oil
10 drops Rose essential oil
10 drops Neroli essential oil
Add to a 4 oz. mister.
Add the essential oils to the mister bottle and then add the water, cap and shake well. Mist your body, or the area around you. I like this blend for alleviating panic.

Dreamtime

10 drops Lavender essential oil

10 drops marjoram essential oil
5 drops sandalwood essential oil
5 drops Ylang,-Ylang, essential oil
5 drops Patchouli essential oil
10 drops Chamomile essential oil
Add to a 4 oz. mister.
Add the essential oils to the mister bottle and then add the water, cap and shake well. Mist your body, or the area around you. I like lightly misting my bed sheets before bed.

Silent Slumber
10 drops Valerian essential oil
10 drops Tangerine essential oil
10 drops Patchouli essential oil
Add to a 4 oz. mister, or use as a diffusion blend, without the water.
Add the essential oils to the mister bottle and then add the water, cap and shake well. Mist your body, or the area around you.

Relax and Let Go
10 drops Tangerine essential oil
10 drops Sweet Orange essential oil
10 drops Patchouli essential oil
10 drops Bergamot essential oil
Add to a 4 oz. mister
Add the essential oils to the mister bottle and then add the water, cap and shake well. Mist your body, or the area around you.
This blend is good for nagging issues and stresses.

Uplifting Blend
20 drops Orange (Citrus sinensis) essential oil
15 drops Grapefruit (Citrus paradisi) essential oil
10 drops Ylang Ylang (Cananga odorata) essential oil
Add to a 4 oz. mister.
Add the essential oils to the mister bottle and then add the water, cap and shake well. This blend is wonderful for when you are feeling tired or needing a lift during the day.

Blends you can make into mists of body sprays.

Anxiety
5 drops Cedarwood (Cedrus atlantica) EO
5 drops Clary Sage (Salvia sclarea)EO
5 drops Tangerine (Citrus reticulata) EO
Or
5 drops Sandalwood (Santalum album) EO
5 drops Frankincense (Boswellia carterii) EO
3 drop Lavender (Lavendula officinalis) EO
2 drops Marjoram (Marjorana hortensis) EO

Fatigue, mental
These blends are helpful for parents. Moms and Dads are often so mentally exhausted, they need a little help sometimes.
10 drops Frankincense (Boswellia carterii) EO
10 drops Lavender (Lavendula officinalis) EO
5 drops Spearmint (Mentha spicata) EO
5 drops Rosemary (Rosmarinus officinalis) EO
5 drops Rosewood (Aniba rosaeodora) EO

Impatience
5 drops Chamomile (Matricaria chamomilla) EO
10 drops Lavender (Lavendula officinalis) EO
10 drops Ylang-Ylang (Cananga odorata var genuina) EO

Insomnia
10 drops Chamomile (Matricaria chamomilla) EO
5 drops Clary Sage (Salvia sclarea)EO
10 drops Lavender (Lavendula officinalis) EO
15 drops Orange (Citrus sinensis) EO
5 drops Sandalwood (Santalum album) EO
10 drops Tangerine (Citrus reticulata) EO
3 drops Ylang-Ylang (Cananga odorata var genuina) EO

Irritability
5 drops Chamomile (Matricaria chamomilla) EO
5 drops Cypress (Cupressus sempervirens) EO
5 drops Lavender (Lavendula officinalis) EO

5 drops Sandalwood (Santalum album) EO

Joy, lack of
10 drops Orange (Citrus sinensis) or Mandarin (Citrus reticulata) EO
10 drops Tangerine (Citrus reticulata) EO
10 drops Grapefruit (Citrus paradisi) EO

Lethargy, listlessness
You can use any with a total of twenty five drops for the blend in the 2 tablespoons carrier oil.
10 drops Clary Sage (Salvia sclarea) EO
10 drops Cypress (Cupressus sempervirens) EO
5 drops Juniper (Juniperus communis) EO
Or
10 drops Lemon (Citrus limon) EO
10 drops Orange (Citrus sinensis) EO
2 drops Rosemary (Rosmarinus officinalis) EO
3 drops Sandalwood (Santalum album) EO

Moodiness, mood swings
You can use any with a total of twenty five drops for the blend in the 2 tablespoons carrier oil.
5 drops Eucalyptus (Eucalyptus globulus) EO
10 drops Geranium (Pelargonium graveolens) EO
10 drops Lavender (Lavendula officinalis) EO
Or
Rosewood (Aniba rosaeodora) EO
Cedarwood (Cedrus atlantica) EO
Clary Sage (Salvia sclarea) EO
Or
Coriander (Coriandrum sativum) EO
Bergamot (Citrus bergamia) EO
Peppermint (Mentha piperita) EO
Vetiver (Vetiveria zizanoides) EO

Nerves, exhausted
Nervous exhaustion is common in this day and age. We are all over-worked, over-tired and striving to get it done. These

blends can help with that. We all have different nervous systems, so find a blend that will work for you.

You can use any with a total of twenty five drops for the blend in the 2 tablespoons carrier oil.

10 drops Chamomile (Matricaria chamomilla) EO
10 drops Clary Sage (Salvia sclarea) EO
5 drops Juniper (Juniperus communis) EO
Or
Lavender (Lavendula officinalis) EO
Marjoram (Origanum majorana) EO
Rosemary (Rosmarinus officinalis) EO
Black Pepper (Piper nigrum) EO
Or
Peppermint (Mentha piperita) EO
Cardamom (Elettaria cardamomum)

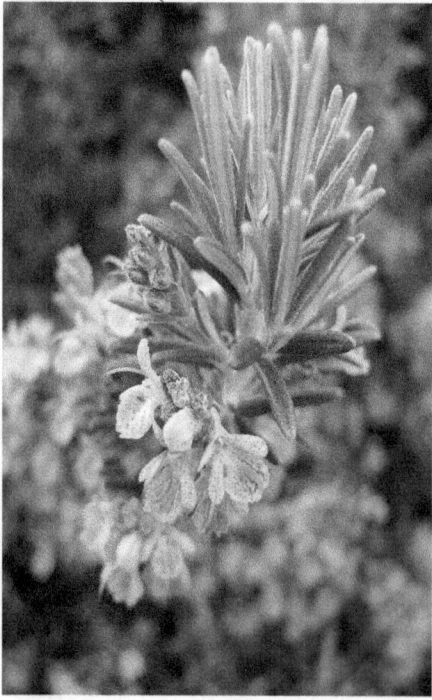

Rosemary (Rosmarinus officinalis) EO
Vetiver (Vetiveria zizanoides) EO
Or
15 drops Basil (Ocimum basilicum) EO
10 drops Pine (Pinus sylvestris) EO
Or
5 drops Pine (Pinus sylvestris) EO
10 drops Rosemary (Rosmarinus officinalis) EO
10 drops Clary Sage (Salvia sclarea) EO
Or
10 drops Peppermint (Mentha piperita) EO

15 drops Lavender (Lavandula angustifolia) EO
Or
5 drops Chamomile EO
10 drops Clary Sage (Salvia sclarea) EO

10 drops Vetiver (Vetiveria zizanoides) EO

Nerves, being nervy
15 drops Chamomile (Matricaria chamomilla) EO
10 drops Juniper (Juniperus communis) EO

Overburdened
15 drops Rosewood (Aniba rosaeodora) EO
10 drops Sandalwood (Santalum album) EO

Overburdened, by responsibilities
15 drops Rosemary (Rosmarinus officinalis) EO

Over-emotional
10 drops Eucalyptus (Eucalyptus globulus) EO
10 drops Ravensara (Ravensara aromatica) EO
Overwork
10 drops Lavender (Lavendula officinalis) EO
15 drops Rosewood (Rosa damascena) EO

Overwork, mental strain from
We all suffer from this at times. It is a balance if being chilled out and stimulated at the same time.
10 drops Clary-sage (Salvia sclarea) EO
15 drops Rosemary (Rosmarinus officinalis) EO

Resentment
Releasing resentment is really hard, we all struggle with these feelings.
This blend is very helpful for this issue.
Make a blend with 20-25 drops of any of the oils below.
10 drops Clary Sage (Salvia sclarea) EO
10 drops Lemon (Citrus limon) EO
Or
10 drops Sandalwood (Santalum album) EO
5 drops Ylang-Ylang (Cananga odorata var genuina) EO
5 drops Helichrysum (Helichrysum angustifolia) EO
5 drops Rose (Rosa damascena) EO

Resentment with Anger
10 drops Grapefruit (Citrus paradisi) EO
10 drops Spikenard (Nardostachys jatamansi) EO
Or
10 drops Yarrow (Achillea millefolium) EO
10 drops Yuzu (Citrus junos) EO

Stress, general- use any of the following essential oils
Just make your blend with a total of thirty drops in your carrier oil.
Cedarwood (Cedrus atlantica), Chamomile (Matricaria chamomilla), Clary Sage (Salvia sclarea), Geranium (Pelargonium graveolens), Juniper (Juniperus communis), Lavender (Lavendula officinalis), Marjoram (Origanum majorana), Tangerine (Citrus reticulata)
You can use these to blend your own stress combating blend.

Stress 1- 20 drops Tangerine (Citrus reticulata), 10 drops Lavender
Stress 2- 10 drops Marjoram, 10 drops Juniper, 10 drops Cedarwood
Stress 3- 10 drops Geranium, 10 drops Clary Sage, 10 drops Chamomile
Stress 4- 5 drops Marjoram, 20 drops Lavender, 5 drops Tangerine (Citrus reticulata)

You can use any of these blend for stress or connected feelings associated with stress.
You can also use these essential oil blend in a liniment for stressed shoulders and sore muscles.
You can use alcohol or witch hazel as your base to put the essential oils in. Do not use robbing alcohol, stick to the beverage variety. 80 proof. If in doubt, use vodka.

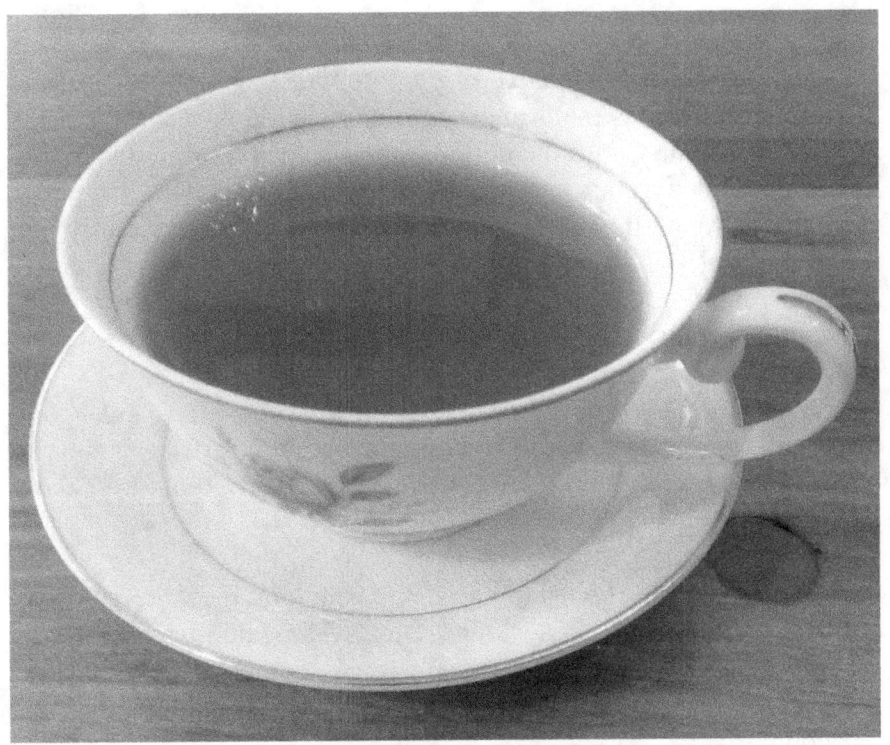

5 HERBAL TEAS

Believe me, I love my cuppa, but medicinal teas and my cuppa are two different beverages. A tea generally steeps until the strength you want it, a few minutes, or while you drink. Medical teas follow the following guidelines.

Infusions

Infusions use the more fragile parts of plants, like leaves and flowers. There are few exceptions to this and Valerian (*Valeriana officinalis*) is one root prepared as an infusion because of its high volatile oil content. This involves pouring boiling water over the plant matter and allowing the matter to infuse. A medicinal infusion steeps for 20 minutes - overnight.

I really like to let my infusions steep for a generous amount of time. I like to allow steeping to occur for about an hour, others only steep for 20 minutes, and it is a personal choice. If it is an herbal tea I really want to enjoy hot I add it to a thermos, or insulated cup to keep it warm.

Decoctions

This is the method used to get the plant healing constituents from more tenacious plant material such as bark, root or nuts. This is simmered gently with the herb in the water for 20 minutes.

For pre-blended roots and leaves the decoction is the preferred method of preparation. The same goes for a decoction: I really like to let my infusions steep for a generous amount of time.

It is really essential to me that they are medicinally potent because I suggest teas for so many tonic and medicinal uses for clients and I want them to work.

Amounts of herb used for decoction or infusion: 1 tablespoon dried herb per cup of water, or two tablespoons fresh herb per cup of water. Teas can be made by the quart and refrigerated for daily consumption.

For teas you will be using parts. A part in any measurement you choose, 1 teaspoon, 1 tablespoon, 1 cup. The catch is for a recipe all parts have to be based on the same measurement.

So if you are using teaspoons then 1 part is 1 teaspoon, 2 parts is 2 teaspoons.

Most teas have a dosage of 1-3 cups a day. Start off with one a day for a week and see if you have any benefits, if not, add another cup week two and repeat for week three. If you have significant benefit with one cup a day, that is wonderful. No need to up your dose with herbs often less is more.

Lemon Stress Tea
1 part Lemon Verbena
1 part Lemongrass
2 parts Lemon Balm
Make as an infusion.
Suggested Dosage: 1-3 cups a day.

Passion Flower De-stress Tea
1 part Passion Flower (Passiflora incarnata)
2 parts Hibiscus Flower
1 part Rosehips
Make as an infusion.
Suggested Dosage: 1-3 cups a day.

L-L-L Stress Tea
2 parts Linden Flower (Tilia spp)
2 parts Lemon Balm
1 part Lavender Flower
Make as an infusion.
Suggested Dosage: 1-3 cups a day.

Daily Toning Tea
1 part Ashwagandha (Withania somnifera)
1 part Holy Basil (Ocimum sanctum)
1 part Rhodiola (Rhodiola rosea)
1 parts Schisandra (Schisandra chinensis)
2 parts Wild Oats (Avena sativa)
Suggested Dosage: 1-3 cups a day.

Morning Stress Buster
1 part Oats, tops (Avena sativa)
1 part Skullcap
1 part Peppermint
2 parts Yerba Mate'
Make as an infusion.
Suggested Dosage: 1-3 cups a day.

Sundown Stress Relief
2 parts Chamomile Flowers
1 part Catnip Leaf (Nepeta cataria)
1 part Skullcap Leaf
1 part Rose Buds
Make as an infusion.
Suggested Dosage: 1-3 cups a day.

Oat More Tea

1 part Oat tops
2 parts Chickweed
1 part Plantain
Make as an infusion
Suggested Dosage: 1-3 cups a day.

Serious Stress Relief
1 part Eleutherococcus senticosus
½ part Valerian Root (Valeriana officinalis)
1 part Hops (Humulus lupulus)
Use before bed and make as a decoction.
Suggested Dosage: 1-3 cups a day.

Rooted and Grounded
1 part Eleutherococcus senticosus
1 part Passion Flower (Passiflora incarnata)
1 part Red Raspberry Leaf
Suggested Dosage: 1-3 cups a day.

MotherStress
1 part Red Raspberry Leaf
1 part Motherwort (Leonurus cardiac)
2 parts Stinging Nettles (Urtica dioica)
Suggested Dosage: 1-3 cups a day.

Floral Stress Tea
1 part Hyssop
1 part Chamomile flower (matricaria recutita)
1 part Feverfew
Make as an infusion.
Suggested Dosage: 1-3 cups a day.

Stress No Stress
2 parts Holy Basil (tulsi) leaf
1 part Lemon peel
1 part Nettle leaf
2 parts Oats
1 part Schizandra berry
Suggested Dosage: 1-3 cups a day.

Sleep the Stress Away
1 part Passionflower leaf (passiflora incarnata)
2 parts Lemon Balm leaf (melissa officinalis)
2 parts Chamomile flower (matricaria recutita)
1 part Licorice root (glycyrrhiza glabra)
Suggested Dosage :Take a cup before bed.

Pumpkin into a Carriage Tea
1 part Dandelion root
1 part Eleuthero root
2 parts Burdock root
½ part Yellow Dock root
This tea is for when your stress is related to overindulging.

You can also make your own tinctures and extracts using these recipes as guides. Page 21.

6 RESOURCES

Herbal Schools
Heart of Herbs Herbal School
501 Lindsey St.
Reidsville, NC 27320
866-303-4372
www.heartofherbs.com
This school is directed by the books author- Demetria Clark

Herbal Suppliers

Mountain Rose Herbs
www.mountainroseherbs.com

Frontier Co-op
www.frontiercoop.com

Starwest Botanicals
www.Starwest-Botanicals.com

Bulk Herb Store
www.bulkherbstore.com

Stony Mountain Botanicals
www.wildroots.com

Fresh Herbs and Seeds

Horizon Herbs
www.horizonherbs.com

Richters
www.richters.com

Essential Oils

Mountain Rose Herbs
www.mountainroseherbs.com

Nature's Gift
www.naturesgift.com

The Essential Oil Company
www.essentialoil.com

Aura Cacia
www.auracacia.com

Swiss Aromatics
originalswissaromatics.com

SunRose Aromatics
www.sunrosearomatics.com

Lab of Flowers
www.labofflowers.com

Carrier Oils

Mountain Rose Herbs
www.mountainroseherbs.com

Frontier Co-op
www.frontiercoop.com

Bulk Apothecary
www.bulkapothecary.com

Essential Wholesale

www.essentialwholesale.com

Herb Seeds

Abundant Life Seeds
www.abundantlifeseeds.com

Johnny's Selected Seeds
www.johnnyseeds.com

Bountiful Gardens
www.bountifulgardens.org

Seed Savers Exchange
www.seedsavers.org

Fedco Seeds
www.fedcoseeds.com

Seeds of Change
www.seedsofchange.com

High Mowing Organic Seeds
www.highmowingseeds.com

Territorial Seed Company
www.territorialseed.com

Bottles and Containers

Cape Bottle Company
www.netbottle.com

SKS Bottle & Packaging, Inc.
www.sks-bottle.com
Also supplies droppers, jars, salves, and tins.

Sunburst Bottle Company
www.sunburstbottle.com

Mountain Rose Herbs
www.mountainroseherbs.com

Great Cape Herbs
www.greatcape.com

Herb and Aromatherapy Associations
American Herb Association
www.ahaherb.com

American Herbalists Guild
www.americanherbalistguild.com

Herb Research Foundation
www.herbs.org

National Association for Holistic Aromatherapy
www.naha.org

United Plant Savers
www.unitedplantsavers.org

ABOUT THE AUTHOR
Demetria Clark lives in NC with her husband, sons, two cats, a dog and frog. She spends her time working at Heart of Herbs Herbal School www.heartofherbs.com and Birth Arts International, www.birtharts.com   She is also the author of Herbal Healing for Children. She believes in love and family first in all things.
Other Titles
Herbal Healing for Children
475 Herbal and Aromatherapy Recipes

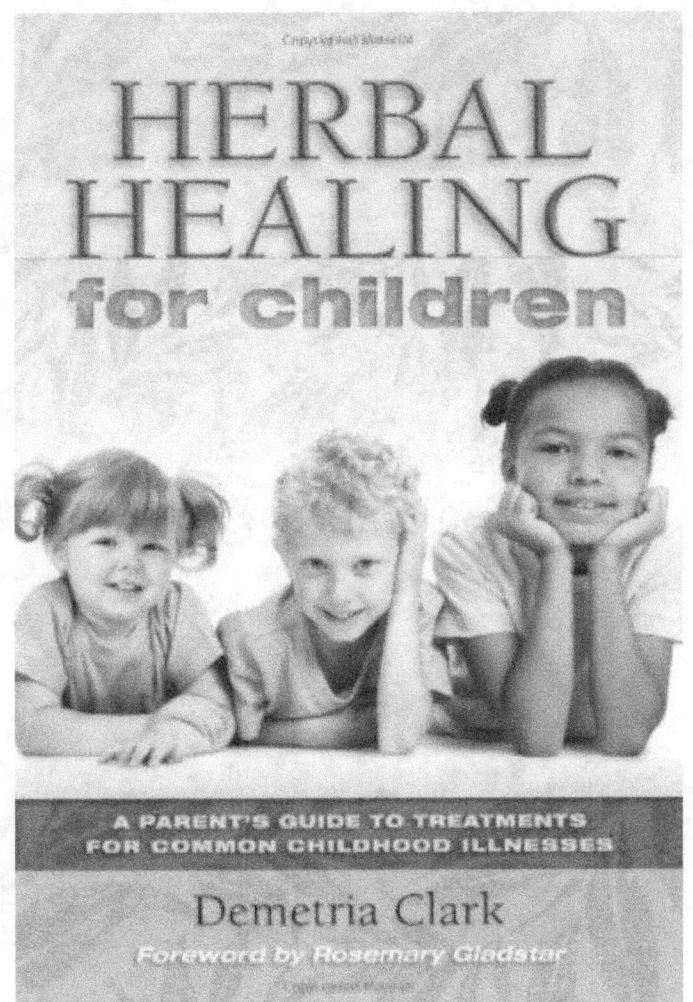

475 HERBAL AND AROMATHERAPY RECIPES

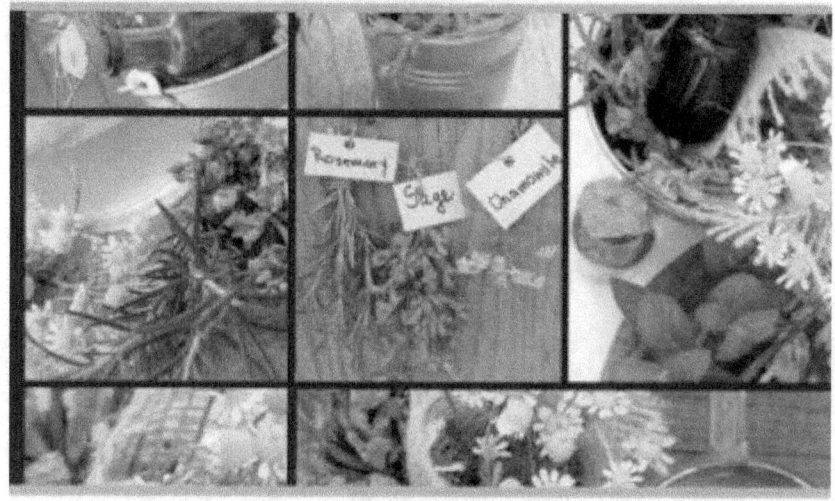

RECIPES FOR LIFE, FAMILY AND ALL OF YOUR HOUSEHOLD NEEDS.

DEMETRIA CLARK

www.ingramcontent.com/pod-product-compliance
Lightning Source LLC
Chambersburg PA
CBHW060220290526
45789CB00003B/1340